Living in the Shadow of Death

Living in the Shadow of Death

A Rabbi Copes With Cancer

Rabbi Stuart G. Weinblatt

Ktav Publishing

Living in the Shadow of Death: A Rabbi Copes With Cancer

Copyright © 2015 by Stuart G. Weinblatt

ISBN 9789655241709

Typeset by Ariel Walden for Urim Publications

Printed in USA

KTAV Publishing House, Inc.
527 Empire Blvd.
Brooklyn, NY 11225
orders@ktav.com
(718) 972-5449
www.ktav.com

Library of Congress Cataloging-in-Publication Data

Weinblatt, Stuart G., author.
  Living in the shadow of death : a rabbi copes with cancer / Rabbi Stuart
G. Weinblatt.
    pages cm
  Includes bibliographical references and index.
  ISBN 978-965-524-170-9 (hardback)
  1. Weinblatt, Stuart G. — Health. 2. Cancer — Patients — United
States — Biography. 3. Rabbis — United States — Biography. 4.
Cancer — Religious aspects — Judaism. 5. Spiritual life — Judaism. I. Title.
  RC265.6.W44 2015
  362.19699'40092 — dc23
  [B]   2015017762

I am extremely grateful to

JACK and JEAN LUSKIN,

and to KEN and STACY SAMET

for their generous help which made publication of
this book possible.

Dedication

I am in awe of the medical profession and of the dedicated men and women who devote their lives to healing and caring. I would not be here were it not for the doctors, nurses and health care professionals who nursed me back to health. They truly are doing God's work. I was fortunate to be under the care of Dr. Bruce Cheson, a brilliant hematological oncologist at MedStar Georgetown University Hospital who administered my treatments and guided the whole process.

I have always felt I am lucky to have such a wonderful congregation, and congregants who are friends. Throughout this ordeal, they were extremely supportive. The genuine concern expressed by so many brought its measure of healing.

Most of all, I thank my family who were so unbelievably loving and supportive. My wife Symcha carried me through it all and was by my side every day. Her love and encouragement eased the burden and pain as she showed me dimensions and depths of compassion which even went beyond the infinite love I had seen in her before.

My children, Ezra, Margalit, Micha and Noam, and son-in-law, Dr. Jason Moche, were truly my dream team. A day did not go by when my children did not call and tell me they loved me. When I lost all my hair they posted pictures throughout the house of other people without hair. They posted articles and notes of cheer on the refrigerator and reminded me of the importance of positive thoughts. Without their love, support and humor I never would have gotten through it all. They gave me what to live for and helped to give me the tools to do so.

Foreword

by Gail Ifshin

IN AUGUST 2010, RABBI STUART WEINBLATT was surprised by a cancer diagnosis.

How could he be sick? His job was to provide comfort to others who are sick or suffering; this could not possibly be happening to him.

But it was. In the chapters ahead, Rabbi Weinblatt chronicles his year of living with cancer. Punctuated by his sermons between Rosh Hashana 2010 and 2011, Weinblatt's narrative deftly weaves together themes of illness and uncertainty with the solace and strength he derives from his spirituality, from Jewish teachings and traditions. Mixed together with a healthy dose of humor, he creates an inspirational account of living from illness to remission.

Indeed, *Living in the Shadow of Death* has a definite emphasis on "living."

Readers need not have experienced serious illness in order to identify with, and gain strength from

Weinblatt's story. His fears, as well as the sustenance he derives from Judaism, are expressed in language that is straightforward and relatable.

In fact, the Jewish teachings and prayers that are so seamlessly a part of his account, equip even the non-observant with a spiritual framework to which they can turn if they someday feel the need (including an appendix of relevant prayers and psalms).

Throughout, Weinblatt emphasizes the importance of appreciating life and its essential components: love, family and community.

Prayer for Weinblatt is not transactional. He does not ask God, as so many of us naturally do when faced by a dire diagnosis, "Why me? Haven't I been good enough?", or ask God for the provision of a cure. Instead, he tells us we have a god that hears our cries. We are not alone. Prayer for him is a link to all who came before and will come after who will turn toward God as a source of solace and wisdom. Rabbi Weinblatt's God is accessible and loving. As is his book.

How It All Began

August 2, 2010

Dear Congregants,

Since I am not sure how best to break the news, or to share with you some personally disturbing information, I will cut straight to the chase.

I am writing to let you know that I have been diagnosed with lymphoma and will begin chemotherapy treatment this Wednesday. I will not know until I meet with the doctor tomorrow what kind of lymphoma it is, but on Friday he concluded, based on the pathological results of a biopsy done last week, that it is best to begin treatment right away.

I have full confidence in the outstanding medical care and attention I am receiving. With trust in the Almighty and Merciful God who watches over all, I hope to have a *refuah shlema*.

I am most appreciative in advance for your prayers and concern for me and my family and am looking forward to celebrating the new year with you and our congregational family in a few weeks.

Your humble servant,

Rabbi STUART G. WEINBLATT

A Surprising Diagnosis

HOW DID I COME TO WRITE THIS LETTER to my congregation and what precipitated it? Around Passover 2006, I had a recurring pain in my back that turned out to be a kidney stone.

When I started having pain in my back again, albeit on a different side four years later, I thought it must be a recurrence of the kidney stone problem. I went to see the same urologist who had treated me previously. I saw his face drop as he reviewed the MRI. Visibly shaken, the doctor, who is a congregant and friend said to me, "You do not have a kidney stone, but there is a growth that wasn't here four years ago."

With those words, a new chapter in my life began to unfold.

Although he used the words growth and tumor, I could not believe what I was hearing. I was certain that there was a smudge mark on the MRI, just as there is sometimes a smudge mark or a thumbprint on a photocopy machine, which then is reproduced onto the copy.

Over the next several weeks, I saw and was referred to a number of doctors who tried to diagnose the cause of my pain, the nature of the growth, and how to treat it. I did not have much of an appetite and was losing weight. Being oblivious to the reality of what was transpiring, I thought I was demonstrating tremendous will power in cutting down on my food intake.

My doctor directed me to a surgeon to see if the growth that was identified on the MRI could be removed surgically. The surgeon said it was in too precarious a place and that I needed to see a kidney transplant specialist since it was so close to the kidney. The kidney transplant specialist wisely advised that before doing any kind of surgery, he wanted to see a biopsy to diagnose the nature of the growth. A week later I had a colonoscopy, and then an endoscopy, during which a tube is inserted through the throat to extract tissue for analysis.

The doctor evaluating the extract said while it was helpful, the sample was not large enough to give a definite prognosis. By now I had a CAT scan and a PET scan, both of which had indicated that the growth was not confined to one area, but that there were a number of microscopic growths in my lungs. I was now under the care of Dr. Bruce Cheson, a hematological oncologist at Georgetown University Hospital.

Originally, the doctor asked me to schedule an

appointment for a bone marrow sample the next week. But, as it was late on a Friday afternoon, he decided to do it right away, rather than delay or wait any longer. Since most of the staff had left already, my wife acted as the "nurse." Having bone marrow extracted is painful. The procedure reminded me of the reverse of "The Matrix" movie, in the sense that something was inserted into the body. I went from there straight to a Friday evening service and barbeque, attended by about 200 people, many of them new and prospective members. I conducted the service, smiling and masking my concern and anxiety, not telling anyone what was going on since I did not have any definitive concrete information about my condition.

Once the results of the biopsies were obtained and the interventional radiologist had extracted additional tissue, the doctor told me it was necessary to begin chemotherapy treatments immediately. Whereas originally he had said that the treatments could begin once I came back from a planned trip to Israel I was leading for members of the congregation, now he insisted that the first treatment needed to begin right away. My wife asked him, "What happens if we wait to begin the treatments after he comes back from Israel, as originally planned?" The doctor responded, "If you wait, based on how fast the tumor is growing and spreading, in two months your husband will be dead."

That certainly got our attention. It was clear we

could not delay. My first treatment was scheduled for the following week.

I sent an email on Friday to the people on the trip saying we would have a conference call on Sunday morning to talk about last minute details associated with the trip, which was scheduled to leave two days later, on Tuesday. When we spoke on the phone on Sunday morning, after going through various matters, I informed the group that I would not be able to travel with them, as I was just diagnosed with non-Hodgkin's lymphoma and that I needed to begin chemotherapy treatments immediately. There was a pregnant pause and silence on the line. I assured them that if it was at all possible, I would join them the week after my first treatment and would be with them for the final part of the trip. People had planned the trip for quite some time, and I knew they wanted to see Israel, but they also wanted to see it with their rabbi. I did not want to let them down. My wife also felt it was important for me to go to the Holy Land and to offer prayers at the Wall.

Once twenty people knew that I had been diagnosed with lymphoma and was going to begin chemotherapy treatments, I knew that the secret would not be contained much longer. That was when I sent the message on the preceding page to members of the congregation informing them of my condition.

Word spread quickly beyond the congregation and in the general community, and evoked a great outpouring of concern. After my first treatment as I lay in the hospital bed still hooked up to the IV, the people in my office told me that they had been inundated with phone calls from members of the congregation asking how I was doing. At that point, as I lay in the hospital bed while still hooked up to the IV, I dictated by phone the following email to the congregation.

Message to the Congregation After My First Treatment

August 4, 2010

In the immortal words of W.C. Fields, "All things being equal, I'd rather be in Philadelphia."

I had the first treatment today and am pleased to report that everything went well and that the doctor and nurse were pleased with the initial results.

Your prayers and good wishes have buoyed me and given me much strength. I appreciate your concern and love.

Stuart D. Weinblatt

Rabbi WEINBLATT

A Change in Scenery

AFTER THE FIRST TREATMENT I FELT TIRED and weak. I had no idea what to expect. My doctor told me that he had a patient who ran a marathon race while undergoing chemotherapy treatment. I was certain I would be that patient who would be able to do the marathon.

I led Shabbat services three days after the first round of chemotherapy. I felt tired, had a bad taste in my mouth, and sucked on a lollipop the whole time.

Although I did not feel well over the weekend and spent most of it in bed, I thought I would still be able to make the congregational trip to Israel I had planned to lead and fulfill my promise to join the group.

There is a Hebrew saying, "*meshaneh makom, meshaneh mazel*: A change in place results in a change in one's mazel, i.e., one's luck." My wife cited this and encouraged me to go on the trip to Israel, as she felt it would be therapeutic to do so.

Five days after the first treatment, a friend flew me up to New York on his private plane so I could then take the international flight to Israel. By the time I got to Kennedy International Airport, I was feeling progressively weaker, tired and uncomfortable. Whereas I usually walk much faster than my wife and have to slow down so that I am not too far ahead of her, as we walked in the airport terminal, I lagged far behind her. I was feeling nauseous, constipated with stomach pains and vomiting.

I took the El Al flight to Israel and slept almost the entire way over.

When I got off the plane, I could barely stand. I had planned to go to the Kotel, the Western Wall, when I got to Jerusalem, to recite prayers with family members. I was feeling very weak and drained. I told the members of my wife's family who came to take me to the Wall, "Instead of going to the Kotel, we have to stay here at the hotel."

After resting up, we joined the synagogue group the following day in Beit Shemesh. Slowly, but surely, I started to feel better. Everywhere we went I received blessings from people – whether they were religious or not. On Friday night at the Wall, I had a most extraordinary experience chronicled here in the sermon I gave a few weeks later on Rosh Hashana evening.

Dancing with Elijah

ALTHOUGH NO BOOK IN THE BIBLE BEARS his name and no writings are attributed to him, there are more legends and stories in Jewish folklore about Elijah than any other Biblical character. Most of us associate Elijah with being a visitor at our Passover seders.

Throughout his life Elijah wandered from place to place, with the Bible saying that he departed from earth in a chariot of fire, borne by a whirlwind up to heaven. His mysterious disappearance gave birth to the popular figure of Jewish tradition and lore created by the rabbis of a person not bound by time or space, who wanders over the face of the earth in a variety of disguises, acting as a celestial messenger. He appears in times of distress and danger, befriending and helping the poor and those in need. He brings consolation to the afflicted. In some stories, he rescues Jewish individuals and sometimes, whole communities. Elijah is regarded as the precursor who heralds the coming of the Messiah, which is why he appears at the Passover seder and is an honored guest at every *brit milah* (circumcision) as well as at the Havdalah ceremony at the end of the Sabbath.

Moving freely about earth unrestrained, without regard to space or time, he takes on disguises as appropriate so that his true identity is hidden. He usually takes the form of a poor person or a beggar, as if to test to see how he will be treated. He rights wrongs by rewarding the poor and punishing the greedy who do not share their wealth with others.

A story in the Talmud places him at the gates of the town sitting with other lepers so they will not be alone and to bring them comfort, disguised as a fellow leper. You can tell the difference, though, because whereas the others bind all the bandages of their sores at the same time, he does so one at a time. The rabbis explain he does it this way so that if he is needed to help another, he will be able to come to their aid unhesitatingly, without any delay.

An example that typifies the many stories about Elijah is of a *yeshiva bachur*, a student who told his father, the *rav*, the rabbi of the town, how much he wished to meet Elijah. The father told his son, "If you study Torah with unceasing devotion you will be worthy of him appearing to you." And so he applied himself with diligence. One night a poor man dressed in tatters wandered into the study hall carrying a heavy pack. The young man turned the stranger away saying the *beit midrash* was not a place for tramps, and so he left. Later his father asked him if anybody had come to visit, and his son told him of the poor straggler he had sent away. Immediately his father said that the visitor was none other than Elijah the Prophet and that he had missed his chance to meet him. For the rest of his life the boy who became a great rabbi in his own right, made a point of saying "shalom" and going out of his way to welcome everyone into his home or place of study.

In a story that has many versions and variations, Elijah disguises himself as a poor wayfarer who is invited to eat a meal by a poor family, even though they themselves have little to eat. Before he leaves to go on his way he tells them he would like to grant them a wish, since they have been so generous even though they have so little. The couple asks to be relieved of their poverty. Many years pass, and the same poor visitor returns and finds that the now prosperous couple has a large home with many servants. When he asks to see them he is turned away by guards. Seeing that the couple has used the wealth he gave them for themselves rather than sharing with others the prophet restores them to their previous status and takes away what he gave to them.

A unifying characteristic of the various stories about Elijah is that the prophet is always anonymous, which brings me to the story I want to share with you.

This August I went to the Wall, the Kotel, in Jerusalem on Friday night a little more than a week after my first chemotherapy treatment. It was crowded, packed with Jews from all over the world decked out in all kinds of dress and costumes and customs. Myriads of *minyanim* were jammed next to each other. Each group had its own way of davening, its own tunes and style. I escorted the people of our group from one side to the other, to expose them to the cacophony of the wondrous sounds and to see and hear, to touch and smell, and to take in all the beautiful ways in which with such joy Shabbat was welcomed and God was praised in His holy city.

After surveying the various groups, we settled upon joining one minyan where the singing was spirited, and they were dancing while singing a *nigun*, a wordless melody that flowed into *Lecha Dodee*. I was happy to be able to be in Jerusalem at the Kotel and to be able to offer my prayers to welcome the Sabbath. Truth be told, I was also thinking a bit about my condition.

And just then, as we were with these strangers, a man with a short white beard, white hair, and a warm smile looked at me. He didn't just look at me. He fixated on me. He pointed to me and picked me out of the whole crowd in the circle. He extended his hands towards me and with a twinkle in his eye, grabbed me, and started to joyously dance with me as the *nigun* was being sung. It was a moment I will never forget.

He danced and prayed with so much fervor, *kavana*

and intent. I felt he wanted me to share in the joy, to feel uplifted, to forget my troubles and to experience joy instead. I couldn't help but wonder, and think to myself: Did this anonymous man somehow know? Did he have any idea what I was feeling and going through? Did he single me out for some reason? Did he know the worries, concern, or anxiety I was feeling at that time?

I have no way of knowing and never will, and I really do not wish to know. For later as I reflected on what happened I thought, perhaps, maybe, just maybe, it was Eliyahu HaNavi, Elijah the Prophet, who came to dance with me and to uplift my spirits. Perhaps it was that anonymous messenger who is sent for any of a variety of reasons to earth by God to help others in time of need.

The High Holiday liturgy quotes the prophet Malachi that the prophet Elijah will not only bring peace, but that he will turn the hearts of parents to their children and of children to their parents. May this new year be one in which we know the blessings of reconciliation, of peace and of joy, the blessings of the prophet Elijah.

Amen.

September 8, 2010

I had been advised about the importance of limiting my exposure to germs. As a result, I did not follow the Torah Scroll and walk through the congregation at Shabbat services. As a way of explanation prior to the High Holidays, I sent the following message to the members of the congregation.

A MESSAGE FROM RABBI WEINBLATT

One of the most enjoyable parts of our holiday services is seeing and greeting friends. And that often entails handshakes, kisses, and a warm hug or embrace. This year, due to my regimen of chemotherapy, I am particularly susceptible to infection, and my doctor has suggested I refrain from coming in close contact with crowds. As a result, please forgive me (and help me) by not giving me a hug or kiss or even shaking my hand at this time, especially if you suspect you may be ill. And believe me, this is one of the most difficult aspects of my treatment!

Your humble servant,

Rabbi STUART G. WEINBLATT

Preparing for "The Sermon"

I KNEW THAT AS WE PREPARED FOR THE NEW year, a little more than a month after my first chemotherapy treatment and about six weeks after the congregation had first learned of my diagnosis, that everyone was concerned and worried and wanted to know how I was doing. I wanted to try and convey a message to the congregation that did not just focus on me. I wanted to take what I was going through and use it as a moment to teach and share how I had drawn upon our tradition and how it had offered me strength and sustenance.

When it was time for the prayer for the sick, the entire congregation spontaneously stood up. Unlike Shabbat when we include the individual names of those who are sick, we do not mention names on the High Holidays since there are so many people. But it was clear that they were all rising in solidarity and concern. I was moved and touched, as were members of the congregation, many of whom were crying and visibly shaken.

To break the tension after the prayer, I said, "This is really something. I am truly touched and overwhelmed. But I must admit, this is quite a way to get a standing ovation."

A little bit later in the service, after the reading of the Torah and Haftara, it was time for me to give my sermon.

Everyone knew what had transpired and could see how I looked. I was thin, pale, and without hair. Many of them were seeing me and my clean shaven head for the first time.

I stood before them, looked out at the congregation, paused and said, "Nu? So how was your summer?"

I then delivered the following sermon.

What Cancer Has Taught Me

Rosh Hashana 2010

A S THE YIDDISH SAYING GOES, "*MENTSCH tracht, und Gott lacht*" – "Man plans, and God laughs."

How true. How true.

I have always thought of myself as healthy, not invulnerable or immune to illness, but as someone with a lot of energy, stamina, and strong willpower. Tumors, a growth, chemotherapy, going bald were all foreign to me. (Ok, three out of four.) Cancer wasn't something that I thought would ever happen to me. It just wasn't in the plan. This was something for which I have offered comfort to others, but I did not think that I would ever be on the other side, the one afflicted with the ailment. Yet *mentsh tracht, und Gott lacht*.

Imagine my surprise when I learned that the pain I was feeling in my back wasn't a kidney stone, as I originally suspected, but a rapidly growing tumor. After a series of tests and many scary, sleepless, worrisome nights when I imagined the worst, I was diagnosed with lymphoma. I was reluctant to ask too much and refrained from getting a second opinion. Perhaps I was afraid I would be told the old Rodney Dangerfield line: "You want a second opinion? You're ugly, too!"

I was and, to be perfectly honest, still am, in a state of shock, finding it hard to believe that this was happening to me. It was all so startlingly new and unexpected. When the doctor told me I had non-Hodgkins lymphoma, I knew so little that I asked which was better: Hodgkins or non-Hodgkins? When he told me, "Hodgkins" I asked, "Can I switch?" As the course and schedule of treatment was being explained to me, I asked the nurse to show me the patient chart. I wanted to be sure the name on the file said, "Stuart Weinblatt." I was in denial. I couldn't believe that the person who was about to undergo a regimen of rigorous chemotherapy was me. The obvious takeaway: listen to your body. If you experience an ongoing unusual pain, do not ignore what your body is telling you. Check it out.

But I want to speak this morning not just about the physical condition, but personally, more personally than I usually do on Rosh Hashana. Not because it's about me, because I know that there are many people who have faced illnesses with direr prognoses and for which the prospects for recovery or successful treatment are not as favorable. Rather, it's about what I have learned from this experience and to share with you what has helped to sustain me through this challenging time, the spiritual dimension. As you can imagine one of my first thoughts when diagnosed during the summer was – I sure hope to get at least one decent sermon out of all of this, for ultimately, the lessons learned parallel and reflect the essential themes of these *Yamim HaNoraim*, the Days of Awe.

Lesson Number One: Be in the moment.

We never know what life has in store for us. One thing though is certain. None of us will live forever, and none of us knows when our number will be up. Think about all the things you want to do, but keep waiting for the right time to do – don't wait too long.

I am reminded of the story told by Rabbi Hayim of Zans about a poor woman who had trouble providing for her many children but was excited, because one day she found an egg and thought all of her problems had been solved. She explained to her children that rather than eat it, she would take the egg and place it under a neighbor's hen so she would then have a chicken. But rather than eat the chicken, she explained she would use it to make and hatch more eggs and chickens, which she will then sell to buy a cow which in turn will yield more cows and calves, which she will use to purchase a field. And as she was proudly dreaming out loud her grandiose plans and feeling so confident in her wisdom and prudence, the egg she was holding fell and broke, shattering all her plans and dreams.

The Hasidic master taught that too often we are like this woman. We allow things to slip away, or through our hands, thinking that we have all the time in the world to do what we intend to do, rather than acting today to use our days wisely to do what we should do and to act on our dreams.

Whatever it may be – that trip to Israel you told me you are going to take one day, that course you have always thought about taking, the hobby you want to learn, spending more time with your children, setting aside time to study, learning a new skill, doing some volunteer work, or even the desire to start attending services more regularly one day, whatever it may be – don't keep putting it off.

I think the central message of the *Unetaneh Tokef* prayer that proclaims that "on Rosh Hashana it is written and on Yom Kippur it is sealed, who shall live and who shall die, who by fire and who by water. . . ." is to force us to come face-to-face with the reality of our mortality. The prayer reminds us of the fragility of life.

Rather than taking it literally, I think the richness of the language lends itself to interpretation and that it was always meant to be understood figuratively, not literally. Hearing it each year summons us to live each moment to the maximum, to recognize that any moment could be our last.

The prayer recognizes that there are some aspects in life that are in our control and for which we determine the outcome. The kind of people we are, the virtues we aspire to acquire, the character traits we seek to live by, what values we embrace, how we respond to the hand that is dealt us – Judaism asserts that these are the kinds of things that are in our grasp and that we can determine. Since we make these choices, our tradition then lays out for us the path we should follow, the things we should try to do, and how to live our lives.

The reason this prayer is so dramatic, powerful, and haunting is because it lets us know that in addition to there being things within the purview of our control and which we decide, there are also those aspects which are truly beyond our dominion. Some events that occur to us are random. Life is comprised of both elements: the things we can affect as well as the unpredicted events, things that happen to us. The point is you never know when to expect the unexpected. Consequently, we live in the crucible of the tension between the two. I have learned that you never know when that unplanned, unanticipated thing will happen, suddenly altering all your plans. One day you are perfectly healthy and the next you find out you have cancer. *Mentsch tracht unt Gott lacht.*

Since as I have now learned firsthand we never know what fate awaits us, which doors are about to open, and which will close, it is important to maximize and enjoy life and every moment as much as possible. My message from my ordeal is that every moment is precious and should be cherished. Take time to appreciate the beauty in our world. Enjoy music, literature, nature, art, the arts – whatever beauty there is all around us, be it created by God or by human beings. There is truth in the old trite adage, "stop and smell the roses." Spend time with the ones you love – now. Don't put off what you have been wanting to do or wait until retirement or some distant elusive moment to begin living.

But at the same time, as much as I advocate for living in the moment and enjoying life, Lesson Number One has an important corollary: Do not live *just* for the moment.

Life that revolves around satiating your own desires and making yourself happy so you will feel good, is ultimately shallow, meaningless, and purposeless. Life needs to be about much more than ephemeral things such as self-aggrandizement, seeking immediate personal gratification, or acquiring material objects you desire. It is most worth living when you live with purpose, when you are connected to something bigger than yourself, such as family, friends, and community, and especially when you recognize and live your life as part of a people that walks with God and as a member of a people who has a mission and purpose.

These two contrasting and conflicting notions, about living in the moment but not just living for the moment, are crucial. If you do one without the other your life is unbalanced and incomplete. Combining the two elements is what puts life into the proper per-spective and makes it worth living.

Rabbi Abraham Twerski writes, "If the purpose of a

human being's existence is contentment, to maximize self-gratification and self-centeredness. . . . God would not have endowed the human being with so superior a mind." He is saying that a mind, like a life, is a terrible thing to waste. We are imbued with intelligence and intellect so we can improve ourselves, so we can do good deeds, make our world a better place, and fulfill God's will, so we can create beauty and develop relationships with others. This is how we find meaning and transcendent lasting values that outlive us.

Our prophets taught us to dream and to work for a better world. Our rabbis introduced the importance of taking responsibility for others and of being a part of a community. Our mystics and later philosophers inspired us not to think only of ourselves, but to work for social justice and equality. Our heritage imposes upon us the imperative and obligation we each have to work for *tikun olam*, to perfect the world. These ideals are some of the finest and noblest gifts bequeathed to human beings.

So while we should live in the moment, do not shortchange yourself by living only for the moment.

In my reading about my disease I came across an anonymous poem entitled, "What Cancer Cannot Do." It goes like this:

> Cancer is so limited . . .
> It cannot cripple love.
> It cannot shatter hope.

It cannot corrode faith.
It cannot eat away peace.
It cannot destroy confidence.
It cannot kill friendship.
It cannot shut out memories.
It cannot silence courage.
It cannot reduce eternal life.
It cannot quench the Spirit.

In many respects in each instance it does the converse, the exact opposite, and strengthens each of these qualities and attributes.

The notion of the spirit, as well as of our obligations and greater responsibilities to others, brings me to

Lesson Number Two: God, faith, and prayer.

There are times during my life when I have been angry with God, when I have argued with God, when I have sought to understand His seeming silence and indifference. I usually feel that way when I see the suffering of others, such as when a family is devastated by a cruel wanton act of terror in Israel, other moments of destruction and devastation or harsh cruelty, when religious fanatics succeed in carrying out plots to kill innocent people in the name of God, or when a young woman who finally found happiness and love is suddenly struck with a fatal illness.

But not this time. I have felt neither anger nor

antipathy towards God as a result of my ailment. I didn't ask, "Why me?" I didn't accuse God of being unfair. Rather, I have found much peace, serenity, and comfort in turning to God in prayer. In part it is because as our tradition tells us, the hand that wounds is the hand that binds. I have prayed the traditional prayers of our liturgy. I have recited psalms and traditional prayers, and I have also expressed the outpouring of my emotions in words and thoughts that I have composed on my own that come from my heart.

The Torah reading for this, the first day of Rosh Hashana, tells us that when Hagar is all alone in the wilderness, God hears the cry of the child, "*ki shema Elohim et kol hana'ar ba'asher hu sham*" – "God hears the child where he is." This is the God I believe in, a God who hears our cries. As Reb Mendel of Worka said when commenting on this verse, "God hears even the silent cries and pleas of the anguished heart, even when no words are uttered."

There were times when I was afraid, especially when the uncertainty of what was the cause of the pains and my loss of weight and appetite weighed heavily on me and my imagination would run wild. I recited then as I do every night the prayer my father would say with me before I went to bed when I was a child. I later learned it was the twenty-third Psalm, "*Adonai roi lo ehzar*" – "The Lord is my shepherd, I shall not want . . . I will fear no evil, for Thou art with me." Saying this prayer implanted and reinforced the belief that God accompanies us, so that even in our darkest moments we are not alone.

Psalm twenty-seven, a psalm we recite at this time of year, affirms: "The Lord is my light and my help, whom shall I fear? The Lord is the stronghold of my life, whom shall I dread? . . . O Lord, when I cry aloud; have mercy on me, answer me. . . . Look to the Lord. Be strong and of good courage."

Our tradition offers a treasure trove of meaningful passages. "*Mima'amekim keraticha*" – "Out of the depths I call You O Lord," "*Esa einai el heharim, me'ayin yavo ezri*" – "I lift up mine eyes unto the mountains, from where will my help come? My help comes from the Lord . . . He will guard you from all harm. . . ." The prayers have been like faithful companions accompanying me along the way. I do not believe that reciting them will change my fate, as if saying them is like waving a magic wand. But praying has brought me solace and reassurance. It has linked me with those of my people who preceded me and those who will come after me who have turned and who will turn to this source of wisdom to find comfort. It makes me feel that I am not alone.

Before each of the operations or treatments, I have said a prayer. I reached out and held the hand of the doctor or nurses, or whoever else was in the room. One of them went something like this:

Ribbono shel olam, Master of the Universe:
Beyadecha afkid ruhi: Into your hand I entrust my fate.

Bezechut avot, Based on the merit of my ancestors, and with trust in You O God who heals the sick, I ask that you guide those who are agents of healing. May I be worthy of a *refuah shlema*, a complete healing, and may my prayers, as well as of those who love and care about me, be answered.

Holding the hands of others brings me to Lesson Number Three: Never underestimate the love and support of one's community, one's family, friends, and loved ones.

I have always felt and thought that I am blessed to have a unique relationship with my congregants and congregation, different than what many of my colleagues have. There is a certain connection and closeness we have, and never has it been more evident than now. I want to take this opportunity to publicly acknowledge and express my gratitude for the outpouring of love and affection, the calls, letters, cards, and emails that I have received from so many of you, most of you – actually from everyone except for . . . , and I have already forgotten his name.

Bruce Genderson, our president, informed me that the Board even passed a resolution wishing me a *refuah shelema* (a speedy recovery). I was especially touched and moved when he told me that the motion passed by an overwhelming vote of seventeen to four, with two abstentions.

In truth, each and every note, call, word of support, visit, or act of kindness has brought its own unique message of encouragement. Do not assume that one can ever receive enough or too much support or comfort, that since others are helping, you are exempt, or that your concern is not appreciated. The Talmud tells us that the mitzvah of *bikur cholim*, visiting the sick, reduces the illness by one-sixtieth. A wonderful story in *Masechet Berachot* of the Talmud is of Rabbi Yohanan who healed people, yet when he was ill, he could not heal himself, for he needed the assistance of others.

In all honesty and not with any sense of false modesty, the outpouring of concern has been gratifying, as I had no idea the extent to which I have been privileged to share and touch the lives of so many. I have learned from the response that Lennon and McCartney were right when they wrote, "and in the end the love you take is equal to the love you make."

In addition to friends, congregants, and members of the community, my family, including my siblings, have shared the concern and anxiety. My children have brought me so much joy and have inspired and motived me to want to live so I will see them continue to grow and flourish. Early on Ezra said to me, "Dad, you have to get better so you can be at Talia's (my one year old granddaughter) bat mitzvah." He then immediately corrected himself and said, "not at her bat mitzvah – at her wedding."

My wife Symcha has been an amazing tower and

pillar of strength. Through her worries and anxiety she has shown so much wisdom and strength as well as genuine unbridled concern and infinite love. The look in her eyes, even the tears she has shed, have shown so much depth and have reminded me of the power and beauty of what it means to be in a loving relationship. It is true that love can grow deeper with the passage of time and in confronting challenges. Before we knew the actual prognosis, and there was a remote possibility that maybe all I had was an infection, I turned to my wife and asked, "Symcha, if it turns out to be nothing, will you promise to still always be this nice to me?"

The truth is that a time like this forces you to think about what is really important in life, what our priorities are, and who and what we cherish the most. We most appreciate those who are precious and dear to us when we think about what life would be like without our loved ones. And that is part of what the High Holidays are meant to remind us of, all of us, as well. This is a time to realize who and what is most important to you. Hold close those you love. Spend time with those you hold dear. And let them know by words and deeds how much you care about them as well as how much you appreciate and love them.

In certain respects we don't really know what we have, what is most precious to us and treasured, until we realize that all is a gift from God and that all that we have is passing and ephemeral, as the Psalmist puts it, "we are like a breath, our days like a passing shadow."

So remember to be good to your loved ones and to take care of each other.

I hope that I am worthy of all the good wishes and prayers said on my behalf. I rescheduled my first and subsequent procedures so that I would be able to attend Wednesday-morning minyan before going into the hospital. As I was about to leave for my first infusion one of our members, Ami Sheintal, said to me, "You know Rabbi, with all the prayers everyone is saying for you, the chemotherapy is really just a supplement."

I cannot help but think how much more I wish I could be there and how much more I wish I would have been there for each and every member who has ever turned to me for comfort, and regret if I have ever disappointed anyone in a time of need. I hope that I will come away from this experience a better person, more sympathetic and empathic to the pains of others. After my first treatment, when I was feeling very weak, I reached out to speak with a colleague who had battled lymphoma just a few years ago. I asked him, "How do you keep hope alive?" I was feeling that down. He said to me, "Stuart, you will come out of this a better person. You will be a better rabbi." Then he added, "And even if you aren't, people will think you are." That is my hope and prayer, to come out of this a better person and rabbi.

So what do I ask for on this New Year? I pray that each and every one of us will be blessed with good health and that the New Year will be one of meaning and fulfillment. As for me, my hope is to have fortitude and strength to face whatever awaits me. I share the simple wish of the Psalmist, "One thing I ask of the Lord, for this I yearn: to dwell in the house of the Lord all the days of my life, to behold the beauty of the Lord, to frequent His sanctuary." (Psalm 27)

That, and no more surprises.

September 9, 2010

The New Normal Sets In

AS THE FALL UNFOLDED AND THE TREAT-
ments were underway, members continued to
ask about my condition. I chose not to do one
of those CaringBridge websites because I thought it
was a bit self-centered and I wanted to maintain some
degree of privacy.

I attempted to continue to maintain as regular a
schedule as possible. The Board was kind enough to
allow me to purchase a reclining chair for my office so
I could rest when I felt tired. People were amazed that
I maintained a regular schedule. What most did not realize was that just about every day I would go home or
into my office and take a nap for about an hour or two.

I continued to teach my tenth grade confirmation
class every Wednesday night. Even immediately after
several hours of chemotherapy treatment, I came di-
rectly from the hospital and explained to the children
that I did this because I wanted them to know how

passionately I feel about Judaism and how seriously I take it. I wanted them to know that it was important enough that I wanted to come and teach them, even though I just had my chemo treatment. I jokingly told them that it was the ultimate "guilt trip" – if they were going to miss a class, they better have a good reason for missing it.

During my time of treatment, the response by members of the congregation was quite extraordinary and gratifying. Many people wanted to bring meals. And even though there were times when I did not feel much like eating, I realized it was important to allow people to do this for us.

Normally my wife and I are on the other side. We are the ones who give and provide for others. It is not in our nature to be the recipients. But I realized it was important to allow the congregation to fulfill the mitzvah for us this time. I sensed that people wanted to feel they were not helpless, but were doing something tangible to express their concern. So we chose not to decline, but to accept the meals and viewed them as expressions of love.

With the passage of several months, my chemotherapy treatments continued. Eventually a CAT scan and a PET scan were taken several months after the last treatment. I anxiously awaited the results and was excited to hear that the tumor had shrunk and that I was in remission.

Upon hearing this news, I sent the following message

to the congregation, inviting them to come to a service at which time I could thank them for all they had done while I was sick and going through the treatments:

January 29, 2011

With gratitude to the Holy One who is the Source of all Healing, I am pleased to let you know that my doctor has told me that my most recent tests reveal that I am in remission.

I am tremendously grateful to you and all who shared in the anxiety and concern felt by me and my family during this time. The thoughts, prayers, and good wishes of our friends and loved ones have meant a great deal to me. I truly believe the expressions of kindness and support helped to carry me and give me the strength and encouragement I needed these last few months while I was undergoing treatment.

There is a wonderful tradition of *"bentshing gomel,"* reciting a prayer of thanks during the Torah reading when one has been sustained after an illness. I would like to invite you to come to services next Saturday, February 5, when I will recite this prayer, and Symcha and I will sponsor a Kiddush in appreciation of my recovery and for all the goodness extended to me and my family.

Your humble servant,

Rabbi Stuart G. Weinblatt

During this service I delivered the following sermon of thanks:

A Sermon of Thanks

I PRECEDED MY ROSH HASHANA SERMON A FEW months ago with a simple question. I asked, "Nu, so how was *your* summer?" By then I had shared with you the news of my diagnosis. Facing the abyss of uncertainty of my prognosis coupled with the fear of the unknown, but with faith in God, I did not know what to expect.

In a similar vein, I ask once again a simple question this morning: Nu, so how was your fall and winter?

In many respects the two questions are bookends. With the passing of these seasons, a period of time which seems like a blur, a chapter in my life has come and gone, and a new page is turned.

I feel like *Avraham Avinu*, Abraham, our patriarch, about whom our Midrash says, transcended to the other side. I feel like one who has had a burden, a heavy weight, taken off of my shoulders. I feel like the children of Israel looking at the *Ohel Moed*, the Tent of

Meeting, when they see that the cloud has been lifted, and they can now move forward.

I feel all of these things, but most of all I feel grateful, grateful to God for restoring me to health, grateful to all of you who have shown so much love, and grateful to my family for all they have done these past few months.

In last week's Torah portion, *Mishpatim*, we read that one who harms another has an obligation to pay for his health care, *ve'rapoh yerapeh*, "he shall provide for healing." This is the justification given in the Talmud by the rabbis that permits us to seek medical care. Even more, Judaism encourages and requires us to seek the best medical care we can get.

There is an old Jewish joke about a man who travels from his shtetl to the big city of Warsaw to see the most famous specialist in the world for his medical condition. After the visit the doctor tells him the charge for the visit, fifty rubles. The man is shocked and objects that the fee is too much, saying he is a poor man who comes from a poor village. The doctor immediately adjusts his rate and says "no problem," he will charge half the amount, twenty-five rubles. The man holds his ground and demands to know how the doctor can in good conscience charge so much for an office visit. Things get progressively unpleasant. After further bickering back and forth, the patient says, "Look doctor. I am not a rich man. I tell you what, I will pay you what I can afford, two rubles, and that's it." The doctor is justifiably upset and asks, "If that is all you can afford, then why did you come to see the most expensive doctor in all of Warsaw?!" And the man says, "Doctor, you don't understand. When it comes to my health nothing is too expensive."

Based on the passage in the Torah as explained in the Talmud, *Masechet Bava Kamma*, our sages conclude that although God is ultimately the healer, we are required to seek remedies for illness. We cannot say, "If God wants me to be ill, I will be ill, and if God wants me to recover, God will heal me without medical intervention." Healing is so important in Judaism that our religion teaches that doctors do the work of God and are partners of the Holy One. No offense to anyone, or what any of us does for a living, but I hope our best and brightest will always aspire to work in the medical profession and that our most caring and compassionate will want to do this work.

I was fortunate to have outstanding medical care. My doctors, David Jacobs, Lenny Bloom, as well as the hematologist who treated and restored me to health, Dr. Bruce Cheson at the Lombardi Center of Georgetown University Hospital and his team, along with the nurses who administered the chemotherapy, are *malachim*, messengers, God's agents of healing.

In a similar vein as in the previous story, a man is given bad news by his doctor who tells him he has only six months to live. The poor guy doesn't know what to say, and then when he gets the bill he says, "This is terrible news doctor. But I must tell you I can't afford to pay your bill, especially not so quickly." So the doctor says to him, "Ok, tell you what, I'll give you a year to live."

I am tempted to go on and continue with a series of medical jokes, but I think you might like to hear something a bit more profound this morning, such as about how I reflect on what I have experienced. Knowing that I have to save a little ammunition for the High Holidays, I still would like to share a few insights with you this morning.

I realize and feel that I was truly blessed to have a network of friends and congregants who shared the experience with Symcha, my children, and me. You were there every step of the way, with cards, notes, and expressions of love. Many of you showed your concern in a number of ways, some by sending or preparing meals, so that Symcha wouldn't have to worry about this. Others conveyed their feelings just by the worry and anxiety I saw in their eyes. To tell you the truth, at first it wasn't easy to be on the receiving end of such generosity, especially for my wife, Symcha, who is such a giving person and who prefers to do for others than to accept any help. But when we saw the outpouring, I began to realize that this was all part of the healing. I realized that we are connected, that we are a community, and that we were in this together. So we learned to be on the other end. And by the way, this is not just about or for me. Even now, one of our beloved members who I visited yesterday, is in the hospital. She knows that she is not alone because she is a member of a community, a caring community.

Knowing that so many prayers were being offered by so many people was truly gratifying and uplifting. At one point I got a little worried that I might be in danger of overdosing on the prayers. Rabbi Nachman of Breslov tells us that humans have the capacity to reach out in three directions – to God, to other human beings, and to ourselves. He taught that when you reach in one of those three, you encounter the other two.

At one time or another, all of us make innocuous comments that we might not really mean. How often do you ask someone "How are you?" and don't wait to listen to the answer. "Have a nice day" is another innocent, harmless, but more often than not, not particularly sincere, comment. When people have a birthday, we wish them a happy birthday and then often add the words, "and many more." When I celebrated my birthday this past December and people wished me a happy birthday and said "and many more," I felt like it had a whole new meaning. I know that it is just a phrase, a throwaway line. But I took it seriously and felt people really meant it.

We Jews have at least three blessings associated with reaching milestones and times of transition. One is on the occasion of the bar mitzvah of a child. Traditionally one says, what is referred to as the *baruch shepetarani*.

The full blessing praises God, "*shepetarani me'onsho shel zeh,*" literally, for relieving a parent for "the punishment for this one." In other words, thank God now that this child of mine has reached the age of majority; I will no longer be held responsible or accountable for his punishment. Now what he does is on his head, not mine.

The other one is the one I said this morning after the Torah reading, *birkat hagomel,* thanking God "*she-gamalani kol tov,*" – "who extends goodness even upon the undeserving." It is a humble expression of gratitude that recognizes that although we may not be worthy, we appreciate being restored to health. The prayer is said on four occasions: completion of long journeys by sea or land, upon release from captivity, and after recovery from a major life-threatening illness. I especially love the translation in the Bokser siddur, as it captures the essence of the emotion one feels at a time such as this:

> Praised be Thou, O Lord our God, King of the universe, who dost shower Thy blessings upon me, even beyond my merits. Thou hast been gracious unto me and hast delivered me from peril. I shall ever praise Thy name and strive to be worthy of Thy continuing love.

I fully identify with this sentiment, which leads me to the third prayer recited when we reach a particular milestone, one that is surely familiar to all of you, the *shehecheyanu* prayer. It is the ultimate prayer of thanks, gratitude for life itself, for being given the gift of reaching a particular time, of experiencing something.

I invite you to join me in reciting these words which express gratitude for reaching this moment: "*Baruch ata Adonai Elohenu Melech HaOlam, shehecheyanu, ve-kiyamanu vehegiyanu lazman hazeh.*" – "Blessed are You O Lord our God, Ruler of the Universe who has kept us alive, preserved us and enabled us to reach this day."

Thank you God, and thanks to each and every one of you for all your love and concern.

February 5, 2011

One year after informing the congregation of my condition and a year after the beginning of my treatment as the new year approached, Rosh Hashana offered a chance to look back and reflect upon what I had gone through and all that had transpired.

I wanted to speak once again from the heart, to share what I had learned and what spiritual and philosophical insights I had gained. Since the High Holidays are a time of reflection and introspection, I wanted to teach one last time not about me, but about how much Judaism, the community, and my faith had helped me get through it all.

What a Difference a Year Makes

Rosh Hashana 2011

W HAT WORDS COULD EVER SURPASS the powerful *Unetaneh Tokef*, the prayer recited during Musaf, which captures the essence of this day. It proclaims the sanctity and nature of this *Yom HaDin*, Day of Judgment, declaring that "On Rosh Hashana it is written and on Yom Kippur it is sealed, who shall live and who shall die, who by fire and who by water . . ." It ranks among the most stirring and poignant prayers ever written. It is more than a prayer. I consider it to be a provocative form of poetic prose that gives me pause every time I read or hear it.

Many of us struggle to understand the premise embedded within it. Some seek to understand what it is supposed to mean and grapple with the text. Others are intimidated by it and find the imagery or theology so awesome as to reject it outright, without dealing with the broader perspective or its underlying concepts.

One thing you cannot do is deny its significance or ignore it. It invites us to be challenged by the concept of confronting our mortality and asserts that we are accountable for how we live our lives.

Its origin is equally mysterious and cloaked in drama. Legend attributes the prayer to Rabbi Amnon who lived in Mainz in the 1200s and who was constantly pressured by the Archbishop to accept Jesus and convert to Christianity. He resisted numerous entreaties to do so, but in a moment of weakness, or, more likely, to get a respite from the persistent pleas and concerned about the safety of his people, he agreed to think about it for three days. He immediately regretted that he had even given the perception that he had entertained the thought of converting, instead of rejecting it outright. He agonized over the possibility that any of his fellow Jews would believe that he had a scintilla of doubt about his faith. When the three days passed he refused to respond to the summons of the archbishop. Just before Rosh Hashana, against his will he was forcibly brought before the Church authorities, where he declared that not only did he refuse to convert, but that he regretted that he had even given the appearance of considering the option. I will spare you the gruesome details of what happened next, other than to say that Rabbi Amnon was brutally tortured and his body mutilated. At home, in excruciating pain and dying of his wounds, the rabbi begged his disciples to carry him into the synagogue, for he could no longer walk because of what had been done to him. He wanted to publicly sanctify God's Holy Name in the presence of the entire congregation. He came and recited the prayer which he had composed, dying as he uttered the final words with his last breath. According to the story as it has been passed down, three days later he appeared to Rabbi Kalonymus in a dream and repeated it, asking that this prayer be recited each year, on the Days of Awe, as it has been ever since.

The prayer is always deeply moving, for it conveys the theme and expresses the mood of the holiday, a time of reckoning, of our need to come face to face with the reality of our own mortality. Each year as I say the prayer and look out at the congregation, I realize there are those who are no longer with us.

There are times when the words take on special meaning. Last year was certainly one of those times.

It is hard to believe that a year ago I stood before you with such anxiety, worries, concern, and a lot less hair. It was for me, and as many of you have told me, for many of you as well, probably the most emotionally charged High Holidays. The intensity of the feeling was especially pronounced and heightened because it was a shared, communal experience. I will always be eternally grateful for the love, support, and kindness extended to my family and me.

I don't think I can top last year, nor for that matter, would I want to. (And yes, this summer was a lot better than last summer.)

So many in the congregation, including young people, have asked me how I processed what transpired. I have been asked what Judaism has to say about all of this, what I learned and discerned, and how my faith helped me, or if it was challenged.

Whereas last Rosh Hashana I stood at the precipice of the unknown and spoke of coping with uncertainty, as well as of my hopes and fears, this year I want to share with you the insights gained having gone through the experience. In so doing I am always cautious when I speak personally, because I hope you realize it is never my intent for it to be about me, but rather what lessons and insights I, as your rabbi and teacher, can share with you that may be helpful and applicable. After all, each person brings with them to synagogue their own dreams and disappointments, their unique joys and sorrows, their particular yearnings and prayers, and thoughts about the situations they are dealing with. As always, I am conscious of this and think in terms of the universal implications that may be of interest and beneficial and of how the wisdom of Judaism can be a helpful beacon and tool to help us face what life has in store for us.

Whenever people confront a life-challenging situation they instinctively wonder and ask, "Why me?" It is a natural question. Given the randomness of the universe, we want to understand if there is any logic, pattern, or reason why things happen.

But I must tell you I am often uncomfortable with

two aspects of the underlying assumption. First, the notion that people assume that they are good, and secondly, that they do not deserve to have anything bad occur to them since they are good people.

Don't get me wrong. It's not that we aren't inherently good. Judaism posits that, but our tradition also wisely counsels that we should have a bit of humility in this regard. We are all basically good, but that should not lead to complacency. We can always improve and be better. The Talmud says that at this time of year, when we are judged, as well as at any given moment, we should consider ourselves as having committed an equal number of *mitzvot* and *averot*. By assuming that our good and bad deeds are in equilibrium, we do not become complacent, nor do we feel overwhelmed. The real intent of this approach is to motivate us to do the right thing the next time we are presented with a choice. There are few who are all good or all bad. Most of us are in the middle. This may be one reason why, as I said last year, I never asked the "Why me?" question. I know I am not perfect or immune from hardship.

Another reason I did not spend much energy pondering "Why me?" could be because I was afraid of what the answer might be.

That may be because I often think of the joke about a poor old woman crying her heart out in the back pew of a church, night and day. She cries out to God and bemoans her circumstances, citing a litany of tragedies that have befallen her. Seeking sympathy, or at least some understanding of her suffering, every day she asks the same question. Looking up at heaven, she explains that she is a good woman and surely does not deserve a life filled with so much pain. As is her custom, she concludes, "Why me, God? Why me?" This goes on for an extended period of time. Finally, one day, a miracle occurs. The heavens open up, and right after she calls out and asks, "Why me?" a voice comes out from above. She is elated. It appears that she is finally going to get her answer. First there is great silence, and then the heavenly voice proclaims loud and clear, "Because you tick me off." So perhaps I did not want to ponder, "Why me?" because I was afraid of the answer. But in all seriousness, even if we received an answer, would it really help?

I have never thought that being a rabbi or doing good deeds shelters or protects me from harm. I did not choose to be a rabbi to earn brownie points or to avoid pain or anguish. Had I wanted to choose an easier, more blissful path, I would have become a shul president.

I subscribe to the notion and suggest that we should strive to do the right thing because it is its own reward. While there very well may be a reward in the next world, *olam haba*, doing good and being good is not like having an insurance policy to protect us so that bad things will not happen to us. Were that the case, we would be acting not out of faith, not out of conviction, when performing a mitzvah, but in pursuit of selfish ulterior motives.

One of the points of the *Unetaneh Tokef* prayer is to recognize that there are three factors that go into why things occur in our world. Some things that happen in life may be preprogrammed and may perhaps even be inevitable. Genes, birth order, where and how we grow up, financial circumstances, as well as a number of other factors over which we have no control, play a role in the direction and path our life will take. Then there is the realm of those things which are just random. For no apparent reason, a person may make a wrong turn that can wind up costing or saving his life. The two realms may converge. Natural disasters, for example are the products of laws of physics and nature. How they wreak their havoc, their impact on victims and affected areas, is, however, random.

While we have virtually no control over these first two dimensions, there is a third dimension: those things in the world that are determined by the choices we make. This is the part of life over which we can exert control and where the choices we make can play a determining role in the outcome of various situations. I believe Rabbi Amnon's prayer teaches that some elements of life are beyond rational understanding and are in the first two categories, while some are within our grasp. Life is the intersection of all three dimensions.

One of my goals on the High Holidays is to convey the concept that Judaism teaches that even though our ability to decisively determine the outcome of events is not absolute, there are things we can affect and influence. Even though the percentage of what we can control may be small, it is significant and potent. We have a say in the direction of our lives, especially in terms of the moral and ethical choices we make. This is why it is so important to study Judaism. It provides the tools that allow us to make proper and good decisions in those areas where we do exert control. For ultimately, these decisions have an impact on us, on those around us, as well as on the kind of world in which we live.

I still believe what I said last year, about the importance of appreciating life. We must live in the moment, but not for the moment. I heard from some people who did things they might not have otherwise done, or that they had put off for a while, as a result of hearing my message last year. Yes, it is true that we never know when our time will be up. This is what I think about every Rosh Hashana when we recite the powerful *Unetaneh Tokef*. The Book of Life is open. We do not know who shall live and who shall die, nor can we know how or when our earthly days will come to an end. All we can be certain of is our mortality. The High Holidays remind us of that so that we will fill our days with meaning and purpose. It is perhaps not coincidental that the cycle of Torah readings at this time of year, from Deuteronomy, tells us, "I set before you this day, the blessing and the curse. *Uvecharta be-hayim*" – "Therefore choose life!"

At the risk of disappointing you, I must tell you that

I did not have any major earth-shattering revelations about the meaning of life. After all, it is not as if I suddenly discovered religion! What I did, however, find was that my religious faith helped me get through some tough times and to cope with what was going on.

I agree with those who say that religion should not be a crutch and believe that the greatest of Jewish philosophers and thinkers would not want us to relate in this manner to our faith. Religion, especially ours, is not some kind of primitive hocus pocus or superstition. It is not a matter of reciting some incantations and then healing magically occurring. Nor should it be a substitute for good medical care. One of the things I love about Judaism is that although it is such an ancient religion, it is so intellectually sophisticated, with a rational and reasonable approach and that embraces modernity.

A fascinating story in the Talmud says that during the time of King Hezekiah people would turn to a Book of Healing to be cured of their ailments. They did it so frequently that that the sages hid the book and forbade its use. They took this action because the people were putting too much faith in it, becoming dependent on shamans, and seeking superficial superstitious treatment rather than turning to doctors for medical care. We recognize that one who heals is God's partner, which is why we are commanded to seek medical care and not to rely on miracles.

I found prayer to be extremely comforting and

powerful. In my personal, private prayers I asked for manifestation of God's mercy and compassion, for health and life. I prayed to be healed so that I would be able to continue to serve God and the Jewish people. I asked for a reprieve for me and for others who were sick and for the welfare of those who offer support for loved ones, for the caregivers who helped sustain me and others, who are agents of healing, God's messengers. I prayed to have the fortitude to cope with what I was dealing with. In retrospect, prayer was comforting, because I found that when I prayed, whether at a minyan in synagogue or when I was by myself, I was not alone. This is what I thought of when reciting the immortal words bequeathed to us by the psalmist, "I shall fear no harm, for You are with me." God accompanies us, even and especially at our darkest moments. It does not mean that He will necessarily intervene, but it gives us the reassurance that we confront life with the endless resource of divine love available to us, if we but access it.

One of my wife Symcha's relatives, who is very religious, suggested an explanation similar to a passage found in the Midrash about our ancestor Ya'akov, Jacob: that God especially desires the prayers of the righteous. I would never put myself in that category, of being among the righteous, but the idea that God desires our prayers is an interesting one. While some might be repelled by this, it was meant to offer comfort. Another person said it allowed me to know how much people cared for me. There is an element of truth in that. While I felt the love and support from so many, I think I would have preferred a roast or a couple of nice emails, and could have done without the chemo. Last year after my first treatment, I travelled to Israel where I met so many people, even folks I did not know, who said they were praying for me. Each helped to lift the burden a bit. Small gestures of kindness do matter and are appreciated.

Not just people who know me, but even people who don't know me and even those who I thought didn't like me wished me well, expressed their concern, and offered good wishes. As a result I came away more certain than ever of how important the love and care shown by friends, loved ones, and even acquaintances can be, for we draw strength from each other.

I also came to understand how important it is that we pay attention not only to the patient, but to the needs of the caregivers as well. They also experience stress and are pulled in many directions, as they live the ups and downs of the loved one for whom they are caring, sometimes, even more so. The truth is that we have it backwards. It is not that we do things because we love someone or for those we love, but rather that when we do things for another human being is when our relationship deepens and we discover the meaning of love.

I come away feeling unchanged in my overall outlook on life. I loved life before and still do. I still feel passionate about my commitment to Judaism and the relevance of our tradition, as it is a wellspring of strength. The first thing we are supposed to say upon waking up in the morning is the line from the siddur, "*Modeh Ani lefanecha Melech Hai vekayam shehehezarta bi neshmati, behemla, rabba emunatecha*." – "I am grateful unto you O living and Eternal King for restoring my soul unto me in mercy. Great is your faithfulness." The *Shulhan Aruch*, the code of Jewish law, says that we should rise up in the morning like a lion. I think it means we should be ready to face the challenge of a new day with fresh energy and vigor.

The question that each of us must confront and which the holidays help us to consider is what will be the nature of the life we live and of the choices we make. How will we use the hours in the days granted us in the coming year?

It is often said that we can only truly appreciate that which we have lost or been deprived of. So I want to tell you what I missed most. Some of you may have noticed that I concluded most benedictions last year with the hope that we each shall know God's greatest gifts, the gifts of health and life.

Believe it or not, I missed not being able to fast on Yom Kippur. Of course, I know that when health is an issue, there is no question what Judaism says. A religion such as Judaism that values life and that seeks to prolong and preserve life obviously dictates that such rules may and should be suspended when one's health is at stake.

A Yiddish short story by David Frishman called "Three Who Ate" is about a community afflicted with cholera. The people in the shtetl were dying and almost literally dropping like flies throughout the summer. When it came time for the High Holidays, the rabbi of the congregation had no choice but to order the people to eat and drink on the holy day of Yom Kippur. He stood before his congregation and expounded upon the verse "I give you the commandments this day, *vehai behem*, so that you will live by them." The rabbi quoted the Talmudic interpretation of the Biblical passage that we are given the commandments so that we may live by them. They are not meant to be an obstacle to life, but are a means to an end, to a fulfilling life. When they threaten one's very existence, it is permissible to suspend them. But his beloved congregants refused to obey his command and continued to fast, even as the deaths continued to mount throughout the day.

Finally with tears in his eyes, seeing he had no choice but to demonstrate by his own actions, along with two other officials of the synagogue, before the congregation on the Day of Atonement he followed his own advice and in the sight of all, said a blessing and ate food. As he did, he cried, "*Baruch shem kevodo*" – "Blessed be the name of the Lord."

I relate to the rabbi's misgivings and reluctance to

violate a commandment. The Talmud decreed that all the *mitzvot* can be suspended to save life, except in three circumstances – being forced to murder another human being, commit idolatry, or commit any prohibited sexual offense. But the truth is we are too willing to abandon our ritual practices, not just in these instances. We rationalize our neglect with the self-serving reassurance that "God will understand," when in reality, our choices reflect and say more about our priorities and values than anything else.

The traditions of our faith are the moorings which anchor us to our past and our future. They are what connect us to our fellow Jews and provide a framework for living. The *mitzvot* are how we live a Jewish life. They are part of what gives us our distinct identity. Without Jewish rituals and customs, we are no different than anyone else. They are what has safeguarded and preserved us as a people and kept us alive. I cannot imagine life without the framework provided by Shabbat, keeping kosher, observing the holidays, and all the other things which so enrich my life and make it meaningful. These practices provide a way to sanctify life. When I observe Jewish tradition I feel connected to God as well as to my people. I feel sorry for all those Jews whose lives are devoid of Jewish practice. As music is often referred to as the soundtrack of our lives, rituals are the soundtrack of our lives as well. We just need to learn the tunes so we can sing its song.

Do you know what else comes to mind when I think about what I missed last year?

I missed terribly not being able to walk through the congregation behind the Torah. More than that, I missed not being able to hug or kiss, to shake your hands, to touch you. And so I thought a lot about the importance of human touch and contact and how important it is. Perhaps this is why before creating Eve, Genesis tell us that God mused, "It is not good for the individual to be alone." Life is to be lived in the presence of and with others.

A story I have told before from the Talmud is of a rabbi who heals others by holding their hand. It is about Rabbi Yohanan who holds the hands of two of his colleagues who are sick on different occasions, and brings them healing. "*Yehav li yadecha*" – "Give me your hand," he says. The story is not about a faith healer, but about the power of human touch and of how much we need others. That is why when he falls ill and is asked why he cannot just heal himself, he demurs, "The prisoner cannot free himself." It means we need each other and can only be liberated from our shackles by the touch of another human being.

Two social psychologists from the University of California-Berkeley, who are both avid basketball players, recently analyzed ninety hours of televised professional play. They looked at every team and every player in the league and concluded that the teams that touch the most win the most. Professor Dacher

Keltner, the author of "Born to be Good: The Science of a Meaningful Life," commented on the finding and said, "Touch instills trust. It contagiously spreads good will. It makes players play better on behalf of each other." Researchers say touch can trigger the release of oxytocin, a chemical that induces trust. It can also light up the brain's reward centers and lower the heart rate. (Although, if touched in certain areas, in a certain way, it could have the opposite result and raise the heart rate.)

The study showed that individual players who touched the most performed the best. Bosh was the second touchiest player in the league and a top performer, according to the findings. Keltner said, "I think it's just all about encouragement. You feel a little better when you make a good play and somebody pats you on the back and tells you, 'Good job.'" And it's not just basketball players who benefit from the human interaction, but all of us. And that is an appropriate thing to consider on the High Holidays. To paraphrase the old AT&T long distance commercial, "Reach out and touch those you love."

So as I stand before you on this Rosh Hashana, I remind you, let us not take life for granted. Each day is a gift from God, as is the presence in our lives of loved ones. Last year I prayed with you the words of the psalmist, "One thing I ask of the Lord, for this I yearn, to dwell in the House of the Lord all the days of my life, to behold His beauty, to pray in His sanctuary" (Psalm 27).

What a difference a year makes! I stand before you on this New Year, filled with gratitude and humility that I am here with you in the House of the Lord. May the new year be one of peace, happiness, and prosperity, and most of all, may it be one of health for each and every one of you and all of your loved ones.

September 29, 2011

One More Thought . . .

THERE IS ONE MORE LESSON I WANTED TO share that I felt I had not emphasized enough the previous two years, and so as part of the message I gave the following New Year I spoke about the importance of the small things in life and how they add up.

I played with the contradictory notion that the little things are important and matter, while at the same time positing that we should not dwell too much on the little things.

A Yiddish story is told about a wealthy man who lived in Eastern Europe. When he died, his life's deeds were placed on the scale by the Heavenly court to judge his behavior and determine the fate of his soul, as is done with any soul. The deeds and misdeeds were placed on the respective sides of the scale, and the scales were tilting on the side of denying his soul the bliss of life eternal. The defending angel assigned to the case consulted his client and asked him if he could think of some deed of kindness he may have done that might have been overlooked, anything even if small, or unintentional, he explained to help bolster his case. The soul thought for awhile and then recalled that many years ago when riding in his carriage his driver heard screams from the roadside. The man allowed his driver to stop and rescue a horse and buggy carrying a family from sinking in quicksand.

The prosecuting angel objected and said that the deed should not be accredited to his account, since he had nothing to do with saving the family. All he did was allow his driver to stop and help. But the judge ruled in his favor, and allowed the deed to be added to the scale. Even with this though, there still were not enough mitzvoth in his account and the scales did not tilt in his favor. The defending angel said that more consideration needed to be given, pointing out that it was not just the entire family, but a horse and a buggy that had been saved as well. With that, slowly, the weight shifted to the positive side, changing the outcome of the court decision and the fate of the soul.

The story teaches that a single act of kindness can have more value than we sometimes imagine. Our deeds add up. The little things we do ultimately become the pattern of how we treat others, and who we are.

Here is an excerpt of the sermon about how to keep things in perspective.

The Little Things Matter

LIKE MANY OF YOU, I SOMETIMES WONDER IF the small things we do for others matter. Do they have any impact or lasting value? Are they noticed, much less remembered? Any doubts I may have had were removed when I was going through my chemotherapy treatments the year before last. I discovered how much each and every small act meant to me. Each gesture of kindness, every expression of care or concern meant a great deal to me and brought me tremendous comfort. What was unanticipated was how many people wanted to do something because they specifically remembered things I had done to help them during a difficult time. I was touched when people mentioned something I had said or done for them, often many years ago. If there is any one thing I took away from what I learned when I went through my illness and recovery it is that the small things in life do matter.

As Richard Carlson, author of the best-selling little book, "Don't Sweat the Small Stuff" reminds us in his subtitle, "it's all small stuff." Carlson writes, "Learning to stop sweating the small stuff involves deciding what things to engage in and what things to ignore. From a certain perspective, life can be described as a series of mistakes, one right after another with a little space in between. And one of the mistakes many of us make is that we feel sorry for ourselves, or for others, thinking that life should be fair, or that someday it will be. It's not and it won't. When we make this mistake we tend to spend a lot of time wallowing and/or complaining about what's wrong with life. 'It's not fair,' we complain, not realizing that, perhaps it was never intended to be."

Our deeds add up. The little things we do ultimately become the pattern of how we treat others, and who we are. As Carlson puts it, "You are what you practice most."

The reality is that life might be a bit more complex, and may not be as succinct and easy to package as, "Don't sweat the small stuff." I suggest keeping the following in mind:

1. Be tireless in your efforts to do small things for others.
2. Be careful of the little things you do that may harm others.

But on the other hand –

1. Let go of and consider insignificant and small the slights or bad things done by others to you.
2. When you do wrong another, don't think that it is inconsequential. Seek amends by doing teshuva and asking forgiveness.

And remember to be appreciative of the little things others do for you.

One of my favorite scenes from Thornton Wilder's classic play, "Our Town" is when Emily who has passed away looks back at her eleventh birthday party exemplifies how important it is to stop and appreciate all the things we so often overlook. The scene is when she is standing on a ladder, looking back and says:

"Oh, Mama, just look at me one minute as though you really saw me. Mama, fourteen years have gone by. I'm dead. You're a grandmother, Mama. I married George Gibbs, Mama. Wally's dead, too. Mama, his appendix burst on the camping trip to North Conway. We felt just terrible about it – don't you remember? But, just for a moment now, we're all together. Mama, just for a moment, we're happy. Let's look at one another. . . .

I can't. I can't go on. It goes by so fast. We don't have time to look at one another. I didn't realize. So all that was going on and we never noticed. Take me back – up the hill – to my grave. But first: wait! Just one more look. Good-by. Good-by world. Good-by Grover's Corners . . . Mama and Papa. Good-by to clocks ticking . . . and Mama's sunflowers. And food and coffee. And new-ironed dresses and hot baths . . . and sleeping, and waking up. Oh earth, you're too wonderful for anybody to realize you.

Do any human beings ever realize life while they live it? – every, every minute?"

Her advice resonates and is consistent with what Carlson advises, "if we would just slow down, happiness would catch up to us." We should use these days to reflect on our blessings, and appreciate both the big and small things in life, as well as reflect on the big and small things we need to change and seek forgiveness for as well. In the end, life is about much more than the frustrations of dealing with poor customer service representatives.

September 18, 2012

Afterword

NOW THAT I HAVE COMPLETED MY TREAT-
ments and am in remission, it seems that
more congregants come to speak with me
about the ordeals they are dealing with, especially
when confronting serious health problems. Perhaps
they assume that I bring a greater understanding of
what they are going through and have a heightened
degree of empathy and sensitivity. I suspect that the
conversations I have in these situations are different
than they were previously because of what I have experienced. I listen to their situation with a sympathetic
ear and an enhanced awareness that comes from having gone through the treatments and the emotional
roller coaster associated with cancer. I try to respond
to their emotional needs and spiritual questions while
providing them with a sense of what to expect will occur physically to them.

Throughout it all, in addition to the power of the

strength and support derived from friends, as I indicated in the pages of this book, I found that reciting prayers and psalms also offered me a great deal of comfort. Some I read at specific times and others randomly. Some I would say in the morning and some in the evening prior to going to sleep.

A Hasidic rabbi who came to visit me told me of a beautiful tradition. He asked me how old I was. I told him that I was fifty-seven years old. He said I should then read Psalm Fifty-Eight each day, which I did.

This, as well as the prayers and psalms that I said regularly, which are traditionally recited when one is ill and which brought me comfort, follow.

Appendix

Psalms and Prayers

CHASTISE ME NOT IN YOUR ANGER, LORD, chasten me not Your wrath. Be merciful to me, for I am weak. Heal me, for my very bones tremble, my entire being trembles. Lord – how long? Turn to me, Lord; save my life. Help me because of Your love. In death there is no remembering you. In the grave who can praise You? Weary am I with groaning and weeping, nightly my pillow is soaked with tears. Grief dimes my eyes; they are worn out with all my woes. Away with you, doers of evil! The Lord has heard my cry, my supplication; the Lord accepts my prayer. All my enemies shall be shamed. In dismay they shall quickly withdraw.

Psalm 6

*

HOW LONG WILL YOU FORGET ME, O LORD?
Forever?
How long will You hide Your face from me?
How long shall I take counsel in my soul, having sorrow in my heart daily?
How long shall my enemy be exalted over me?
Look and answer me, O Lord my God!
Lighten my eyes, lest I sleep the sleep of death.
Lest my enemy say, I have prevailed against him;
and those who trouble me rejoice when I am moved.
But I have trusted in Your loving kindness –
my heart shall rejoice in Your salvation.
I will sing to the Lord, because He has dealt bountifully with me.

Psalm 13

*

THE LORD IS MY SHEPHERD; I SHALL NOT want.
He makes me lie down in green pastures.
He leads me beside still waters.
He restores my soul.
He leads me in the paths of righteousness for His Name's sake.

Even though I walk through the valley of the shadow of death,
I will fear no evil, for You are with me –
Your rod and Your staff comfort me.

You prepare a table before me – in the presence of my enemies.

You anoint my head with oil – my cup runs overs.

Surely goodness and loving kindness shall follow me all the days of my life;

. . . and I will dwell in the house of the Lord forever.

Psalm 23

*

THE LORD IS MY LIGHT AND MY HELP. WHOM shall I fear?

The Lord is the strength of my life. Whom shall I dread?

When evildoers draw near to slander me, when foes threaten, they stumble and fall.

Though armies be arrayed against me, I will have no fear.

Though wars threaten, I remain steadfast in my faith.

One thing I ask of the Lord, for this I yearn: To dwell in the House of the Lord all the days of my life, to behold His beauty, to pray in His sanctuary.

He will hide me in his shrine, safe from peril. He will shelter me beyond the reach of disaster.

He will raise my head high above my enemies. I will bring Him offerings with shouts of joy, singing, changing praise to the Lord.

O Lord, hear my voice when I call; be gracious to me, and answer.

It is You that I seek, says my heart. It is Your Presence that I seek, O Lord.

Hide not from me, reject not Your servant.

You have always been my help, do not abandon me. Forsake me not, my God of deliverance.

Though my father and mother leave me, the Lord will care for me.

Teach me Your way, O Lord; guide me on the right path, to confound my oppressors.

Abandon me not to the will of my foes.

False with nesses have risen against me, people who breathe out lies.

Mine is the faith that I surely shall see the Lord's goodness in the land of the living.

Hope in the Lord and be strong. Take courage, hope in the Lord.

Psalm 27

*

A PSALM OF DAVID, A SONG FOR THE DEDI-cation of the temple. I extol you, O Lord. You raised me up. You did not permit foes to rejoice over me.

Lord, I cried out and You healed me. You saved me from the pit of death.

Sing to the Lord, you faithful, acclaiming His holiness. His anger lasts a moment; His love is for a lifetime.

Tears may linger for a night, but joy comes with the dawn.

While at ease I once thought: nothing can shake my security.

Favor me and I am a mountain of strength. Hide Your face, Lord, and I am terrified.

To You, Lord, would I call; before the Lord would I plead.

What profit is there if I am silenced, what benefit if I go to my grave?

Will the dust praise You? Will it proclaim Your faithfulness?

Here me, Lord. Be gracious, be my help.

You turned my mourning into dancing. You changed my sackcloth into robes of joy that I might sing Your praise unceasingly, that I might thank You, Lord my God, forever.

Psalm 30

*

MIGHTY ONES, DO YOU REALLY DECREE what is just? Do you judge mankind with equity? In your minds you devise wrongdoing in the land; with your hands you deal out lawlessness. The wicked are defiant from birth; the liars go astray from the womb. Their venom is like that of a snake, a deaf viper that stops its ears so as not to hear the voice of charmers or the expert mutterer of spells.

O God, smash their teeth in their mouths; shatter the fangs of lions, O Lord; let them melt, let them vanish like water; let Him aim His arrows that they be cut down; like a snail that melts away as it moves; like a woman's stillbirth, may they never see the sun!

Before the thorns grow into a bramble, may He whirl them away alive in fury.

The righteous man will rejoice when he sees revenge; he will bathe his feet in the blood of the wicked. Men will say, "There is, then, a reward for the righteous; There is, indeed, divine justice on earth."

Psalm 58

*

O UT OF THE DEPTHS I CALL TO YOU; LORD, hear my cry, heed my plea.
Be attentive to my prayers, to my sigh of supplication.

Who could survive, Lord if You kept count of every sin? But forgiveness is Yours, that we may worship You.

My whole being waits for the Lord, with hope I wait for His word.

I yearn for the Lord more eagerly than watchmen for the dawn.

Put your hope in the Lord, for the Lord is generous with mercy.

Abundant is His power to redeem; He will redeem the people Israel from all sin. *Psalm 130*

At nighttime I was especially mindful of saying the "Hashkeivenu" prayer, as well as the Shema.

HELP US, OUR FATHER, TO LIE DOWN IN peace; and awaken us to life again, our King. Spread over us Your shelter of peace, guide us with Your good counsel. Save us because of Your mercy. Shield us from enemies and pestilence, from starvation, sword and sorrow. Remove the evil forces that surround us, shelter us in the shadow of Your wings. You, O God, guard us and deliver us. You are a gracious and merciful King. Guard our coming and our going, grant us life and peace, now and always. Praised are You, Lord, eternal guardian of Your people Israel.

*

This prayer from the morning liturgy was also very comforting.

I AM GRATEFUL TO YOU, LIVING, ENDURING King, for restoring my soul to me in compassion. You are faithful beyond measure.

Master of all worlds! Not upon our merit do we rely in our supplication, but upon Your limitless love. What are we? What is our life? What is our piety? What is our righteousness? What is our attainment, our power, our might? What can we say, Lord our God and God of our ancestors? Compared to You, all the mighty are nothing, the famous nonexistent, the wise lack wisdom, the clever lack reason. For most of their actions are meaningless, the days of their lives emptiness. Human preeminence over beasts is an illusion when all is seen as futility.

But we are Your people, partners to Your covenant, descendants of Your beloved Abraham to whom You made a pledge on Mount Moriah. We are the heirs of Isaac, his son bound upon the altar. We are Your firstborn people, the congregation of Isaac's son Jacob whom You named Israel and Jeshurun, because of Your love for him and Your delight in him.

Therefore it is our duty to thank You and praise You, to glorify and sanctify Your name. How good is our portion, how pleasant our lot, how beautiful our heritage. How blessed are we that twice each day, morning and evening, we are privileged to declare:

HEAR, O ISRAEL: THE LORD OUR GOD,
THE LORD IS ONE.

Praised be His glorious sovereignty
throughout all time.